YOUR KNOWLEDGE HAS VALUE

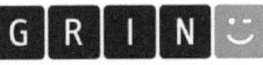
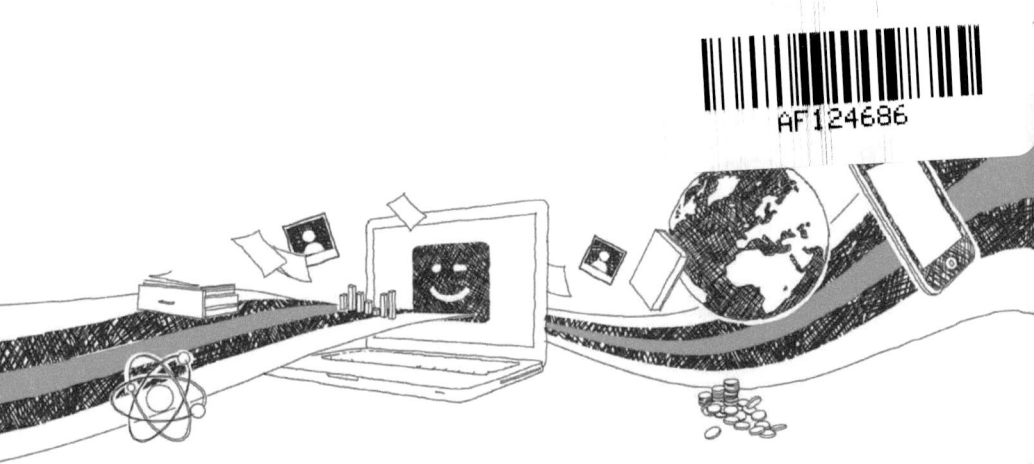

Dr.Sumita Agarwal

The Study of Cephalic Index Of North Indian Students In TMMC & RC

GRIN Publishing

Imprint:

Copyright © 2013 GRIN Verlag GmbH
Print and binding: Books on Demand GmbH, Norderstedt Germany
ISBN: 978-3-656-74733-8

This book at GRIN:

http://www.grin.com/en/e-book/280294/the-study-of-cephalic-index-of-north-indian-
students-in-tmmc-rc

GRIN - Your knowledge has value

Since its foundation in 1998, GRIN has specialized in publishing academic texts by students, college teachers and other academics as e-book and printed book. The website www.grin.com is an ideal platform for presenting term papers, final papers, scientific essays, dissertations and specialist books.

Visit us on the internet:

http://www.grin.com/

http://www.facebook.com/grincom

http://www.twitter.com/grin_com

THE STUDY OF CEPHALIC INDEX OF NORTH INDIAN STUDENTS IN TMMC&RC

BY

DR. SUMITA AGARWAL (BDS)

Research Project being carried in

Teerthanker Mahaveer University, Moradabad (U.P)

MASTER OF SCIENCE

IN

MEDICAL ANATOMY

DEPARTMENT OF ANATOMY

TEERTHANKER MAHAVEER MEDICAL COLLEGE & RESEARCH CENTRE

MORADABAD (U.P)

2011-2012

TABLE OF CONTENTS

LIST OF TABLES

LIST OF FIGURES

LIST OF ABBREVIATIONS USED

CI	**Cephalic Index**
NORMSDIST	**Normal cumulative distribution for the Specific mean and standard deviation**
No.	**Number**
Min.	**Minimum**
Max.	**Maximum**
S.D.	**Standard Deviation**

INTRODUCTION

Cephalometry is the scientific measurement of the dimensions of head.[1] The name Cephalometry is grain to the morphological study of all structures present in the human head.[2] Cephalometry is a branch of Anthropometry.[3]

Anthropometry may perhaps be most simply and comprehensively defined as the conventional art or system of measuring the human body and its parts. The systems of measuring the skull and the skeleton are known separately as craniometry and osteometry, but these terms are frequently merged with that of anthropometry ;thus we speak only of anthropometric instruments, anthropometric methods in anthropometric laboratories.[4]

HISTORICAL REVIEW

Cephalic index was first identified by Swedish Professor of Anatomy Anders Rezitus (1796-1860). With the passage of time constant changes occurred in the structural appearances of human life as *evolution*. Evolution is defined as *genetic change overtime*. CHARLES DARWIN defined evolution as *"Descend with modification"*. Anthropology is a science founded on evolutionary principles.[3] Cephalic index is the term used in anthropology to find out racial differences, sexual differences which are of great significance in diagnosing medico legal cases of forensic medicine.

Man is fond of making comparison to prove his superiority over the increasing size of Phylogeny. Measurements serve as an important guideline for Comparison. Comparative changes in the cephalic index between parents, offspring, and siblings towards their genetic transmission of inherited characteristics.[5]

To compare skulls of different races and species, the physical anthropologist takes various measurements of skull. This process is called Craniometry.[6] The breadth/length ratio is the cranial index (cephalic index in the living). Distinction between measurement of dried crania and living heads, by the two sets of terms, is not rigidly applied. The "Cephalic" terms are more common, often used for both the purposes.[7] internationally accepted techniques of craniometry/Cephalometry have promoted a large number of comparable data for males and to lesser extent, females.

Measurements are important tools for comparisons. Measurements of the body were begun and are used by the artisan, and by the artist, the object of the one being a proper "fit' and that of the other a correct or artistically superior production. They were and are employed in recruiting armies, with the aim of eliminating the inferiors. They are used to some extent by medical men and dentists, to assist them in reaching diagnosis or tracing improvement in their patients. They enter largely into the modern systems of college and other gymnastics, and lately also into those of the popular baby studies. Certain measurements play important role in criminological and medico-legal identification. Finally, we have measurements that have become invaluable aids to scientific research in physiology, anatomy and especially anthropology.[4]

Cephalometry is an important tool for an Anthropologist and Forensic expert for identification of the racial differences, sexual differences, comparison of changes between parents, offsprings and siblings towards their genetic transmission of inherited characteristics and also in forensic practice where cranial remains were compared with existing photographic and radiographic records in identification of disputed identity.[8]

Race: "Biological grouping within the human species distinguished or classified according to genetically transmitted differences". Thus, race is a population concept. Races are populations, which differ in the frequency of some genes.[9]

The population of world is divided into 3 types of races namely[9]:-

1. Caucasians or Caucasoids
2. Mongolians or Mongoloids
3. Negros or Negroid

Table No. 1 – Differentiating features between races [9]

DIFFERENTIATING FEATURES BETWEEN RACES			
FEATURES	**CAUCASIANS**	**MONGOLIANS**	**NEGROS**
COMPLEXION	Fair	Yellowish	Black
FOREHEAD	Raised	Inclined backward	Small compressed
FACE	Small	Large & flattened	Jaw projecting, malar bone prominent
SKULL SHAPE	Rounded	Narrow & Elongated	Square
SKULL LENGTH	Long to short	Long	Long
SKULL BREADTH	Narrow to broad	Narrow	Broad

Table No. 2 – Differences in skull types for determination of races [9]

TYPE OF SKULL	CEPHALIC INDEX	RACE
DOLICHOCEPHALIC	70-75	Pure Aryans, Aborigines, Negroes
MESATICEPHALIC	75-80	Europeans, Chinese
BRACHYCEPHALIC	80-85	Mongolian

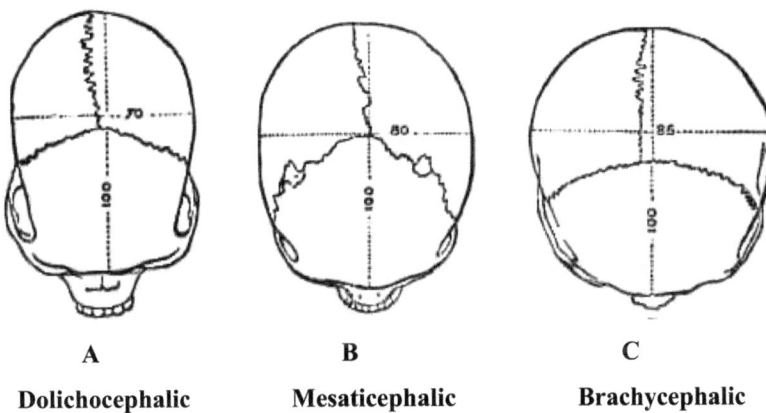

A	B	C
Dolichocephalic	**Mesaticephalic**	**Brachycephalic**

Fig. no. 1 - Showing differences in skull types for determination of races Dolichocephalic skull (Fig. no. 1 - A)

Source: Raveendranath V. & Manjunath K. Y.; An anthropometric study of correlation between cephalic index, cranial volume and cranial measurements in Indian cadavers; *Indian Science Abstracts*; Sep. 2010: vol. 15 (ii); pp. – 55-58.

If the maximum width of cranium is less than 75% of its maximum length, it is called as Dolichocephalic skull.[6]

Mesaticephalic skull (Fig. no. 1 - B): - If the ratio between maximum width of cranium and maximum length of cranium is between 75% to 80%, it is called as Mesaticephalic skull.[6]

Brachycephalic skull (Fig. no. 1 - C): - If the maximum width of cranium is more than 80% of its maximum length, it is called as Brachycephalic skull.[6]

The length and breadth are measured by spreading calipers, and not by measuring tape.

The skull of an Indian is Caucasian with few Negroid characters.From the various measurements of the skull , race can be determined in 85% to 90% of cases. Because of the racial mixing , all the skulls may not be correctly differentiated into the 3 races. Racial mixing has been and is constant and as such pure races are uncommon.

The Mongoloids includes native Americans, Asiatic orientals such as Korean, Japanese, Chinese and Southeast Asians. Most Europeans skulls fall into Mesaticephalic group.

SEXUAL DIMORPHISM: It is generally less marked in mankind than in some other primates. This is to be associated with the paedomorphic tendency of the human stock , not in females but also males being less divergent in adult development , from their juvenile form , than is the case among some other primates , especially in the males.(Abbies 1952; Schultz 1956).

Even in extinct species of mankind sexual dimorphism appears - (on the slender fossil evidence available) - to have been less than in primates.

In modern man the differences are further reduced but the degree of divergence between the sexes in cranial dimensions and proportions varies in different racial groups.

These sexual differences have attracted less exact evaluation than have general studies of ethnic variations.

In both cases, assessment depends upon observation of 2 kinds of features:

- Those which cannot be measured. (Size of mastoid process, prominence of chin).
- Those which are customarily expressed as actual measurements or indices. (eg. Cranial capacity , orbital index)

Craniometric methods have a special usefulness in forensic practice where cranial remains can be compared with existing photographic and radiographic records in making an identification. They also play a part in attempts to reconstruct the appearance in life of Indus represented only by skeletal remains.

The most important of Cephalometry dimensions are length and breadth of head that with them determine the cephalic index. *The Cephalic index is the ratio of the maximum breadth of head to its maximum length.*

CEPHALOMETRY

1. (A) Maximum length of the head, or the maximum antero-posterior diameter; c.e. This is the maximum glabello-occipital diameter of the vault.

Landmarks:

Anteriorly — the most prominent point of the glabella;

Posteriorly — the most prominent point on the occiput as shown by the Maximum determinable spread of the branches of the spreading calipers.

1. (B) The Iniac antero-posterior diameter (optional); c.e.

Taken in the sagittal and median plane of the vault.

Landmarks:

Anteriorly — the most prominent point of the glabella;

Posteriorly — the inion, the individual peculiarities of which should be discounted.[2]

2. The maximum breadth of the head or maximum lateral diameter; c.e.
This is the greatest horizontal and transverse diameter which can be found on the vault by the spreading callipers.

Landmarks:

Determined solely by the maximum breadth of the skull above the supra-mastoid and zygomatic crests.

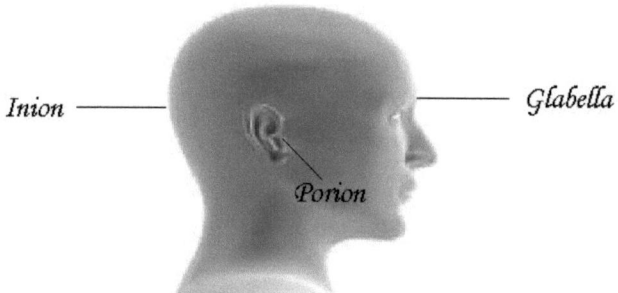

Fig. no.2: - Showing the head points used for the measurements

Source: Raveendranath V. & Manjunath K. Y.; An anthropometric study of correlation between cephalic index, cranial volume and cranial measurements in Indian cadavers; *Indian Science Abstracts*; Sep. 2010: vol. 15 (ii); pp. – 55-58.

REVIEW OF LITERATURE

Cephalic index is an important parameter in evaluating racial and gender differences. A large body of evidence shows a clear racial variation in cephalic index. Therefore detailed knowledge of the population specific data on biometric features of the cranium is important in the study and comparison of the crania of populations from different racial backgrounds, assessing growth and development of an individual and in the diagnosis of any abnormalities of cranial size and shape.[12]

Cephalic index was first identified by Swedish Professor of Anatomy Anders Rezitus (1796-1860) and first used physical anthropology to classify ancient human remains found in Europe.[13]

S. Bharati et al (2001) investigated the relationship between head form and climatic variation in different tribal and caste populations of India. The magnitude of the cephalic index varied significantly in different zones. In tropical zones, head form was longer (dolicocephalic), but in temperate zones, head form was more round (mesocephalic or brachycephalic), especially among Scheduled Tribes (ST) and Scheduled Castes (SC) than among other castes. The authors concluded that these trends possibly support a climatic adaptation model in head form differences among ST and SC in India.[14]

Shah G. V. & Jadhav H.R. (2004) measured cephalic index in medical students of Gujarat, 500 medical students were measured for head length & head breadth and cephalic index was calculated. After comparing previous records of cephalic index with their work, a tendency was proved towards brachycephalisation – an evidence of continuous growth of brain more in the lateral direction. The authors also concluded that the sex as well as race of the deceased can be determined accurately with the head measurement. [15]

Hossain Golam M. D. et al (2005) found secular changes in head dimensions of Japanese adult males. The subjects for the study were all of Japanese birth and Japanese ancestry. The age range of the subjects was between 18 and 25 years. Four head measurements were taken: head length, breadth, height and circumference. In addition, stature and body weight were also measured. All measurements were made by one observer (Fumio Ohtsuki) from 1998 to 2001. The study sample was compared with the series taken between 1910 and 1917 of Matsumura and the one measured in 1965 of Morita and Ohtsuki. The study demonstrated the presence of larger means for head length, head breadth and cephalic index in the current sample than in their predecessors of about 35–85 years ago. Also, the findings displayed larger head circumference than that of the Morita and Ohtsuki series. When ANOVA test was applied for statistical analysis of data, head length and head breadth showed significant ($p<0.01$) differences among all birth-year cohorts from 1978 to 1983 of the current sample. Head height, head circumference and cephalic index did not display significant differences. However, the slope of the regression line indicated that all measurements as well as the cephalic index showed slightly decreasing tendencies during the investigated period. The results suggested that brachycephalization has been occurring for approximately about 35–85 years in adult Japanese males, but the change seems to have become reversed slightly during the period covered by this study sample. [16]

Lobo S.W. et al (2005) found cephalometric characteristics and gender differences in Cephalic Index of a Gurung community, Nepal. Head length, head breadth and Cephalic Index were determined for 267 subjects of Gurung village. The mean Cephalic Index for male was 83.1 and for female 84.6 which

14

was statistically significant. The author concluded at the end of the study that on comparing the results with the existing literature the Gurung community can be categorized as Brachycephalic. [17]

Golalipour M. J. (2006) stated that cephalic index and head shape are affected by geographical, gender, age, racial and ethnic factors. This study was carried out to determine cephalic index and head shape in 410 normal 17- 20 years old female (Turkman group – 200 and Fars group – 207) in Gorgan north Iran. After observing his results and comparing with other studies in the world, he concluded that ethnic factor affects the head dimensions. [18]

Vojdani Zahra et al (2009) conducted the study for determining normal range of head shapes in 867girls and 960 boys in the age of 14-18 in fars-Iran. In regards of cephalic index their results showed that dominant type of head in girls was brachycephalic with 42.5% and in boys was hyperbrachycephalic with 34.3%, rare type of head shape in girls was dolicocephalic with 4.80% and in boys was 7.5%. There was significant difference between boys and girls cephalic index. [19]

Oladipo G. S. et al (2009) determined the cephalic indices among Ogonis. 800 subjects comprising 400 male and 400 female with age ranging from 25 – 45 years, of Ogoni ethnic group by both parents and grandparents, were measured. The subjects were measured for head length and head breadth and cephalic index was worked out by dividing the head breadth by head length and multiplying by 100. The cephalic indices were calculated and the result analysed using Z test. The test analysis indicated that there was significant difference between Ogoni males and females. They also observed that cephalic index is an important parameter for classifying populations. [20]

Odukuma E. I. et al (2010) involved 699 (male – 361, Female – 338) volunteer students of Delta State University whose age ranged around 18 years and over in their study. Respondents were selected along three ethnic groups including Urhobo (male – 156, Female – 147), Ibo (male – 141, Female – 145), and Edo (male – 64, Female – 46). The mean cephalic index (CI) between the randomly sampled populations was 77.95 ± 4.34 cm. There was an observed significant effect of age on cephalic index ($p < 0.01$) but gender showed no significant effects on cephalic index. The values for the three selected tribes did not differ significantly from one another nor differ from the population mean ($p < 0.05$). The mean male and female Cephalic Index values were 77.67 and 78.14 cm, respectively. The Cephalic index patterns of three indigenous West African ethnic groups (Urhobo, Edo and Ibo) were presented in this study highlighted certain features common to West African and perhaps African populations. It was shown that Cephalic index is a significant index for differentiation of population groups and cultures. In spite of these observations, differences which enable intracultural differentiation commonly occur as exhibited by the craniometric pattern in this study. Therefore, authors quoted that craniometric studies are most essential in the study of population dynamics especially with respect to quantitative variables. [21]

Mahajan Anupama et al (2010) undertook the study to document the cephalometric characteristics and gender differences in cephalic index of Punjabi community. Head length, head breadth and cephalic index were determined for 400 medical students (17 – 23 years) of Punjab. After comparing with previous workers it was found that Punjabi community can be categorised as Brachycephalic / Hyperbrachycephalic. This study strengthened the hypothesis that cephalic index is useful in differentiation of racial and sexual differences. [22]

Oladipo G. S. et al (2010) aimed to determine the cephalic length, cephalic breadth and cephalic index of the Ibibios of Nigeria. The study was carried out using 800 subjects of Ibibios who were between the ages of 18 – 80years, comprising of 400(four hundred) males and 400(four hundred) females. The subjects which were Ibibios by both parents and grandparent were randomly selected. The cephalic length (CL), cephalic breadth (CB) and cephalic index (CI) were determined using standard methods. The data obtained showed that the mean values of the CL, CB and CI were 19.06±0.77cm, 15.20±0.71cm and 79.85±4.05 respectively for males and 18.80±0.77cm, 14.70±0.67cm and 78.36±6.12 respectively for the females. The CI shows that Ibibio males and females belong to the mesocephalic group. The mean value of CL, CB, and CI for Ibibios (male and female) were 18.93±0.79cm, 14.95±0.73cm and 79.11±5.24 respectively. Statistical analysis using z-test indicated that significant difference exists between the males and the females with males showing higher values in all the parameters (p<0.05). [23]

Raveendranath V. & Manjunath K. Y. (2010) worked out on 93 formalin fixed cadavers (64 male and 29 female) to find out the correlation between the cephalic index, cranial volume and cephalometric measurements using cadaver heads, observing head length, breadth, and height. The mean cephalic index for male was 76.97 and for female 79.23. With the results they classified the head shapes as Mesocephalic. A positive correlation between cephalic index and cranial volume was found in both sexes. [24]

Adejuwon S.A. et al (2011) examined the cranial indices of 85 skulls recovered from cadavers sourced from South-western regions of Nigeria, mainly populated by Yoruba ethnic tribe. The cranial indices were determined by measuring the maximum cranial length (mcl) and maximum cranial breadth (mcb) using Goniometer fitted with sliding callipers. The cranial index was determined by finding the percentage of the ratio mcb to mcl x100. The skulls were deemed from adult & elderly individuals because of their complete teeth eruption and obliteration of sutures. Gross sexual dimorphic characteristics such as size and overall expression of cranial features (pronounced mastoid process, strong brow ridge) were used to divide skulls into 56 males and 29 females. The mean cranial indices for male and female skulls examined were 72.97±2.16 and 71.72±2.48, respectively, thus placed them in the dolichocranic population. There were no significant differences in the cranial indices of the male and female skulls (p>0.05). Thus cranial index was not sexually dimorphic in the studied skulls. [25]

Jadhav H. R. et al (2011) correlated his study with the data of cephalic indices of various communities of world to understand the geographical influence in altering head dimensions. A total of 180 subjects of six different Communities (30 subjects per community) were selected from the various districts in different regions of Gujarat state, India. The communities were: Sindhi, Patel, Rabari, Kharwa (fisherman), Bhil and Siddi(negro). Only male subjects who belonged to 21 – 50 years of age and who were not having any history of inter-caste, inter-religion marriage of their parents uptill at least 3 generations were included. The study subjects were divided into 3 age related groups: Group A: 21 to 30 years, Group B : 31 to 40 years and Group C : 41 to 50 years. 30 subjects, 10 per aforesaid age-groups (A, B and C) were studied from each community. This was followed by head measurements i.e. head length and width were obtained from each study subject (total being 180) and by cephalic index of each study subject was determined by Hrdlicka's method. The data were then analyzed by statistical software and to determine statistical significance chi-square and Kruskal Wallis tests were applied. The results showed that the value of mean cephalic index in the present study (80.20) was close to the observations made by Shah et al in 2004 in Gujarat, by Bhargav and Kher in 1961 in Barelias and by Oladipo and Olotu in 2006 in Ijaw males. [26]

Maina M.B. et al (2011) studied the different head types in three ethnic groups of North-Eastern Nigeria residing in Gombe. Cephalic length, width and height in Fulani, Tangale and Tera ethnic groups were linearly measured in a total of 322 (152 males and 170 females) 18-40 years old subjects. The result revealed no significant difference in cephalic indices, except in Fulani males, where transverse cephalic index was higher than in the other ethnic groups ($p<0.05$) and in Tangale females where all the cephalic indices were higher than in other ethnic groups ($p<0.05$). Head types based on the indices in males and females from all the three ethnic groups were dominantly High Hypsicephalic and Acrocephalic and rarely Chamaecephalic and Tapeinocephalic according to vertical and transverse cephalic indices, respectively. The study revealed that the three ethnic groups share differences on the basis of cephalic indices and share some similarities on the basis of head types and that Nigerians share similarities with Sri Lankans base on their head types. [27]

Anitha M.R et al (2011) included 100 (64 males and 36 females) north Indian students from different colleges in the age group of 17 to 20 years, to determine the cephalic index. Maximum breadth of the head and maximum length of the head were determined by spreading calipers. Measurements were taken with the subject sitting in relaxed condition and head in Anatomical position. Mean Cephalic Index among males was 79.14, in females it was 80.74. This showed that there was no significant gender difference in the Cephalic Index in subjects from northern regions of India. Northern regions showed predominance of mesocephlaic phenotype in both the sexes. [28]

Ilayperuma Isurani (2011) took a total of 400 subjects with an age span of 20-23 years to establish the cranial indices and head shapes in an adult Sri Lankan population. The cranial length, breadth and auricular head height of the subjects were recorded using a digital sliding caliper and Todd's head spanner. The

19

horizontal, vertical and transverse cephalic indices were calculated using external dimensions of the skulls. There were significant gender differences in all principal cranial dimensions. The mean horizontal, vertical and transverse cephalic indices were 78.54, 78.68 and 100.52 respectively. The predominant cephalic phenotype of the study subjects were brachycephalic, hypsicephalic and acrocephalic. Among males dolicocephalics and among females brachycephalics dominated. The results of this study highlighted the racial and gender differences in cranial morphometry and cephalic indices in an adult Sri Lankan population. [12]

Salve Manoharrao Vishal et al (2011) carried out the study with 320 (160 male & 160 female) medical students of Dr. Pinnamaneni Siddhartha Institute of Medical Sciences & Research Foundation and Dr. Sudha & Nageswara Institute of Dental Sciences Chinnaoutpally, Krishna District (AP), INDIA. The mean cephalic index was 76.94±2.53. The mean cephalic index for male was 75.68±2.05 and for female was 78.20±2.33. The difference between male and female cephalic index was significant (p= 0.001 & difference 2.52). The result of the study showed that majority of male of Andhra region were dolicocephalic or mesocephalic and female were mesocephalic. Cephalic index of the female was 2-3 point higher than the male in Andhra region population. [29]

AIM & OBJECTIVE

To study the sexual and racial variations in cephalic indices of north Indian students in Teerthanker Mahaveer University. Cephalometry is the scientific measurement and morphological study of all structures present in human head which is an important tool for an Anthropologist and Forensic expert for identification of the racial differences, sexual differences, comparison of changes between parents, offsprings and siblings towards their genetic transmission of inherited characteristics and also in forensic practice where cranial remains were compared with existing photographic and radiographic records in identification of disputed identity.

MATERIAL AND METHOD

A total number of 800 Students (400 male & 400 female) of Teerthanker Mahaveer University were examined for this study as they were of cosmopolitan origin, ranging from age group of 17 – 25 years.

INSTRUMENT:-

Measurements were taken with the help of "SPREADING CALIPERS".

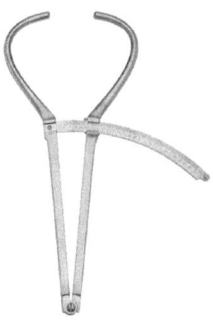

Fig. No. 3 - SPREADING CALIPERS

(Spreading calipers with rounded ends, the tips are made to touch the cranial points and the reading is observed on the scale.)

METHOD:-

With the help of **"SPREADING CALIPERS"** Cephalic Index was measured with the method named ***Hrdlicka's method.***

Cephalic Index is the *head length* (maximum anteroposerior diameter) measured from *Glabella* (point above the nasal root between the eyebrows and intersected by mid sagittal plane) to *Inion* (the tip of external occipital protuberance) and the *head breadth* (maximum transverse diameter) measured between the *Porion* (point on the posterior root of the zygomatic arch above the middle of upper border of external auditory meatus) of each side.

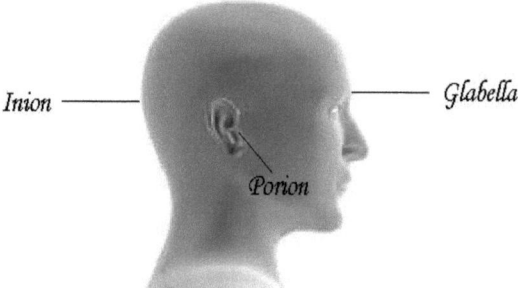

Fig. No. 4 - Showing the head points used for the measurements

Source: Raveendranath V. & Manjunath K. Y.; An anthropometric study of correlation between cephalic index, cranial volume and cranial measurements in Indian cadavers; *Indian Science Abstracts*; Sep. 2010: vol. 15 (ii); pp. – 55-58.

The measurements were taken with the student sitting in the chair, in relaxed condition and the head in anatomical position.

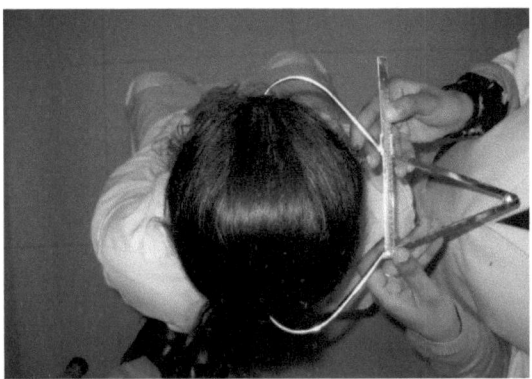

Fig. No. 4 - Showing the measurement of maximum length with the help of Spreading Calipers

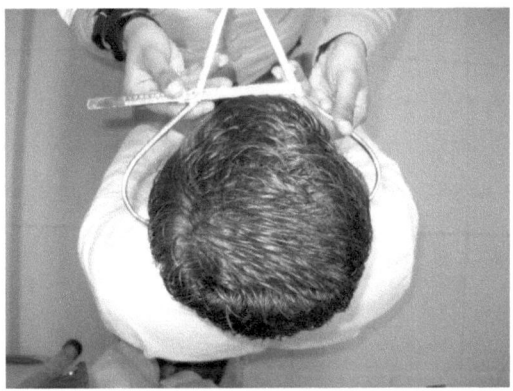

Fig. No. 4 - Showing the measurement of maximum breadth with the help of Spreading Calipers

Cephalic Index was computed by the following formula:-

$$\textbf{Cephalic Index (C.I.)} = \frac{\text{Maximum head breadth}}{\text{Maximum head length}} \times 100$$

OBSERVATION

In present study of comparison of the mean of:-

      a. Maximum Length of Head,

      b. Maximum Breadth of Head and

      c. Cephalic Index.

between the male and female subjects, rests on the following facts.

    1.   The number of both male and female subjects was 400 each.

    2.   As such the total sample size was 800.

The above three different means between the male and the female were compared using Z test for equality of the two means. The Z test was applied because, the total sample size was 800 & as such it is a large sample case. It was assumed that the samples were collected from a normal population whose parameters were unknown.

Hence the Z test was applied as under:-

$$Z = \frac{(\bar{X_1} - \bar{X_2})}{\sqrt{(\frac{\sigma_1^2}{n_1} + \frac{\sigma_2^2}{n_2})}}$$

Where:

$\bar{X_1}$ = mean of sample 1/ group 1 i.e. male subject,

$\bar{X_2}$ = mean of sample 2/ group 2 i.e. female subject,

σ_1^2 = variance of sample 1/ group 1 i.e. male subject,

$\sigma_2{}^2$ = variance of sample 2/ group 2 i.e. female subject,

n_1 = number of units in sample 1/ group 1 i.e. male subject,

n_2 = number of units in sample 2/ group 2 i.e. female subject,

Which follows a standard normal distribution. It is also to be noted that two tail test @ a 5% level of significance was applied. It is known that @ 5% level for two tail the critical value of $Z = \pm 1.96$.

In the present study following statistical formulae were also considered:-

1.   Mean   = $\dfrac{\sum_{i=1}^{n} x_i}{n}$

2.   Variance   = $\dfrac{\sum_{i=1}^{n}(x_i - \bar{x})^2}{n}$

3.   Standard Deviation   = $\sqrt{Variance}$

4. The p value of the Z statistics of all the test have been calculated by using the NORMSDIST function in Excel, which otherwise is not possible.

5. Some other helpful functions in Excel in our calculations, were also worked out, the details of which shall not have any material impact on the actual findings.

Table No. - 3: Statistics of various parameters of present study

Variable	No.	Min.	Max.	Mean	S.D.	Z value	P value
Cephalic index (male)	400	68.50	88.34	79.15	4.06	9.4940	0
Cephalic index (female)	400	72.43	90.62	81.66	3.39		
Cephalic index (male & female)	400	68.50	90.62	80.41	3.95		
Head length of male (in cm.)	400	15.50	20.50	18.51	0.80	18.9886	0
Head length of female (in cm.)	400	14.40	19.50	17.53	0.63		
Head length of male & female (in cm.)	400	14.40	20.50	18.03	0.87		
Head breadth of male (in cm.)	400	13.00	16.40	14.63	0.65	7.2250	5.01
Head breadth of female (in cm.)	400	13.10	16.50	14.32	0.53		
Head breadth of male & female (in cm.)	400	13.00	16.50	14.48	0.61		

Table No. - 4: Classification of subjects based on cephalic index

Sex	No.	Dolicocephalic	Mesocephalic	Brachycephalic
Male	400	68	141	191
Female	400	10	94	296
Total	800	78	235	487

Bar diagram showing classification of subjects based on cephalic index

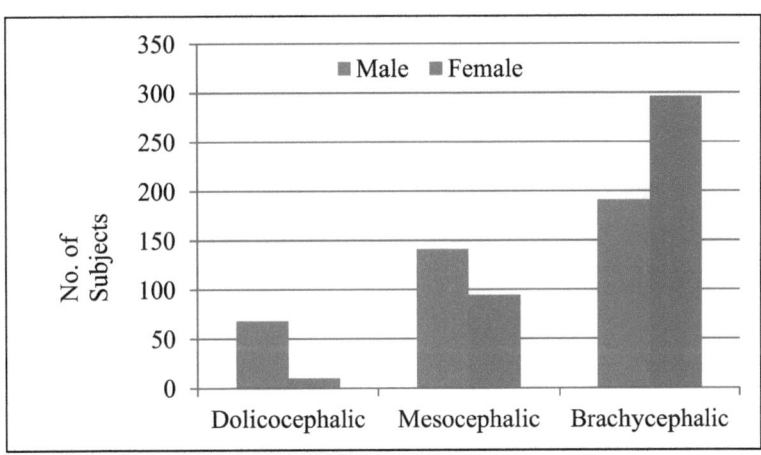

Table No. 5: - Relationship of Sex with Cephalic Index

Cephalic Index	Male	Female	Total
68.00 – 68.99	2	0	2
69.00 – 69.99	6	0	6
70.00 – 70.99	6	0	6
71.00 – 71.99	4	0	4
72.00 – 72.99	13	2	15
73.00 – 73.99	24	4	28
74.00 – 74.99	13	4	17
75.00 – 75.99	25	15	40
76.00 – 76.99	22	15	37
77.00 – 77.99	29	24	53
78.00 – 78.99	33	22	55
79.00 – 79.99	32	18	50
80.00 – 80.99	37	42	79
81.00 – 81.99	48	67	115
82.00 – 82.99	24	62	86
83.00 – 83.99	43	36	79
84.00 – 84.99	22	27	49
85.00 – 85.99	9	21	30
86.00 – 86.99	4	17	21
87.00 – 87.99	2	9	11
88.00 – 88.99	2	4	6
89.00 – 89.99	0	9	9
90.00 – 90.99	0	2	2
Total	400	400	800

Table No. 6: - Head length in males and females

Head Length (in cm.)	Male	Female	Total
14.00 – 14.99	0	1	1
15.00 – 15.99	1	3	4
16.00 – 16.99	8	49	57
17.00 – 17.99	76	220	296
18.00 – 18.99	190	120	310
19.00 – 19.99	107	7	114
20.00 – 20.99	18	0	18
Total	400	400	800

Bar diagram showing head length in males and females

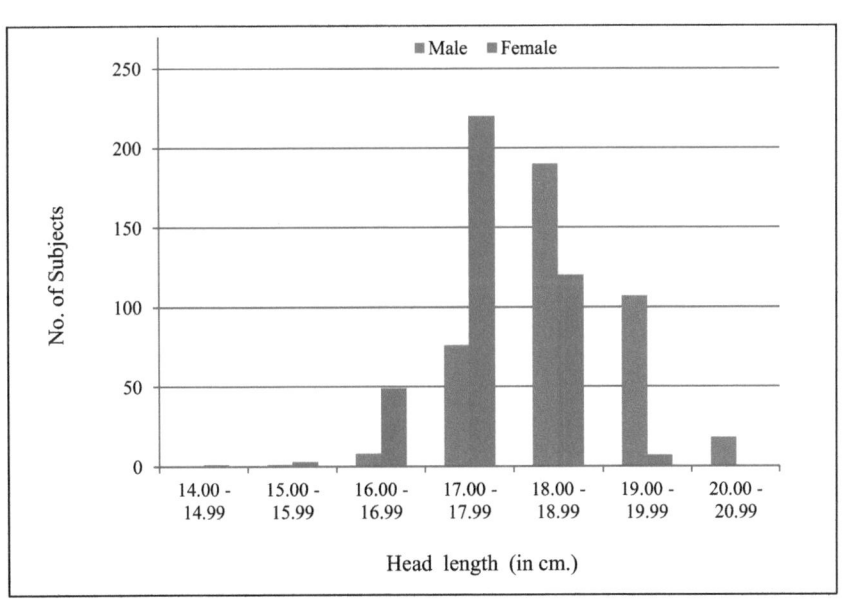

Table No. 7: - Head breadth in male and female

Head Breadth (in c.m.)	Male	Female	Total
13.00 – 13.99	55	72	127
14.00 – 14.99	207	276	483
15.00 – 15.99	127	49	176
16.00 – 16.99	11	3	14
Total	400	400	800

Bar diagram showing head breadth in male and female

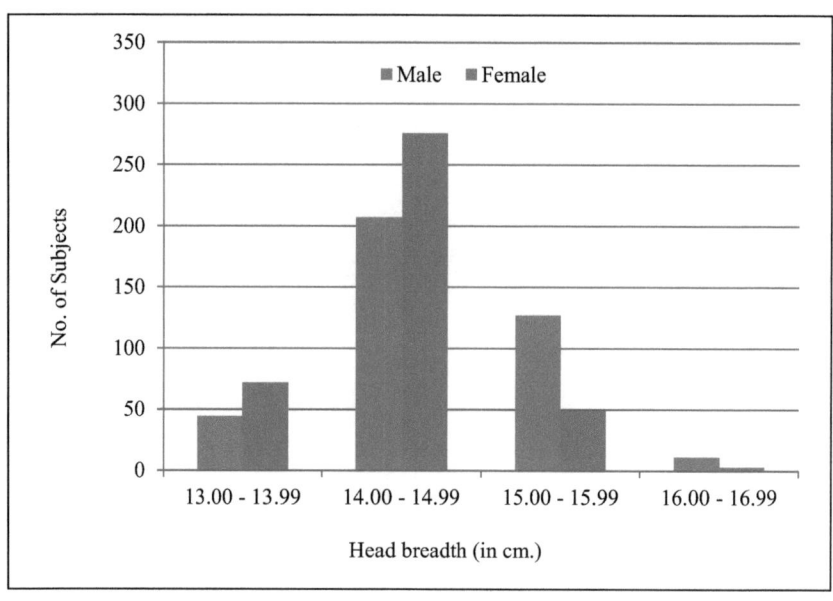

DISCUSSION

The present study provides valuable data pertaining to the cephalic index and shapes of the heads in an adult north Indian population. It is stated that the racial characters are best defined in the skull (Oladipo *et al.*, 2009; William *et al.*). As a result cranial morphometry, and hence the cephalic index constitute the most important diagnostic tool for determining the racial difference (William *et al.*).

Diverse craniometric approaches have been proposed and utilized to estimate the cranial capacity either on dry skulls or living subjects (William *et al.*). During the course of this study cephalic indices were estimated based on the linear dimensions of the skulls. The cephalometry provides a reliable, relatively easy and quick method. Furthermore, this approach has the added advantage as it does not require any sophisticated techniques. Cephalometry continues to be the most versatile technique in the investigations of the craniofacial skeleton (McIntyre & Mossey, 2003; Vojdani *et al.*, 2009).

In present study effort has been made to find the head shapes of the population with the available data in relation to the cephalic index. Total of 800 students have been examined, 400 male and 400 female, ranging from age group of 17 – 25 years.

In the following section the result of the present study when compared with that of previous ones show the following results.

The **mean head length of male** students observed by Shah in Gujarat region is 18.26, by Mahajan in Punjab region is 18.58, by Salve in Andhra region is 18.28 and that by Isurani in sri Lankan populaion is 18.05. In the present study it is 18.51 that coincides with the above – mentioned values. The range in the present study lies within a common range as the previous studies (refer table no. 8).

The **mean head length of female** students observed by Shah in Gujarat region is 16.5, by Mahajan in Punjab region is 17.92, by Salve in Andhra region is 17.26 and that by Isurani in sri Lankan populaion is 17.5. In the present study it is 17.53 which is in conformity with the observations in the previous studies except in Gujarat region. The **range** in the present study as well as previous studies lie within a common range (refer table no. 9).

The **mean head breadth of male** students in Gujarat region is 14.56, in Punjab region it is 15.68, in Andhra region it is 13.82 and that in Sri Lankan population is 14.78. Whereas in the present study it is 14.63 which is coinciding with Gujarat region and Sri Lankan population but higher than Andra region and lower than Punjab region. In the present study the **range** lies within the range of previous observations (refer table no. 10).

The **mean head breadth of female** students in Gujarat region is 14.1, in Punjab region it is 14.72, in Andhra region it is 13.49 and that in Sri Lankan population is 14.11. Whereas in the present study it is 14.32 which is showing a wider value of correlation with previous studies. In the present study the **range** is 13.10 – 16.50, which lies within the range of previous observations except in Andra region where it is higher than that (refer table no.11)

The **mean cephalic index of male** students observed by Shah in Gujarat region is 80.42, by Mahajan in Punjab region is 81.34, by Salve in Andra region is 75.68 and that by Isurani in sri Lankan populaion is 78.04. In present study it is 79.15 which is lower than by observations of Shah and Mahajan but higher than by Salve and Isurani. In the present study the **range** is 68.50 – 88.34 which does not coincide with the values of previous studies where it is lower than Gujarat & Punjab region and higher than Andhra region (refer table no. 12).

The **mean cephalic index of female** students observed by Shah in Gujarat region is 81.20, by Mahajan in Punjab region is 85.75, by Salve in Andra region is 78.20 and that by Isurani in sri Lankan populaion is 79.32. In present study it is 81.66 which is in conformity with the value of Shah's study but lower than by observations of Mahajan and higher than by Salve and Isurani. In the present study the **range** is 72.43 – 90.62, coincides with the observations of shah and Mahajan except the values of Salve's study where it is higher than that (refer table no. 13).

The **mean cephalic index of total** students in Gujarat region is 80.81, in Punjab region is 85.53, in Andra region is 76.94 and that in sri Lankan populaion is 78.54. In present study it is 80.41 which is in conformity with the value of Gujarat region but lower than by observations of Punjab region and higher than by Andra region & Sri Lankan population. In the present study the **range** is 68.50 – 90.62, coincides with the observations of Gujarat and Punjab regions except the values of Andhra region where it is higher than that (refer table no. 14).

Table No. 8 - Comparison of present study with the other studies for head length of male students

Studies	Range	Mean
Shah G.V.	16.5 – 20.1	18.26
Anupama Mahajan	14.01 – 21.92	18.58
Salve Vishal Manoharrao	17.3 – 20.3	18.28
Isurani Ilayperuma	–	18.05
Present Study	15.50 – 20.50	18.51

Bar diagram showing comparison of present study with the other studies for head length of male students

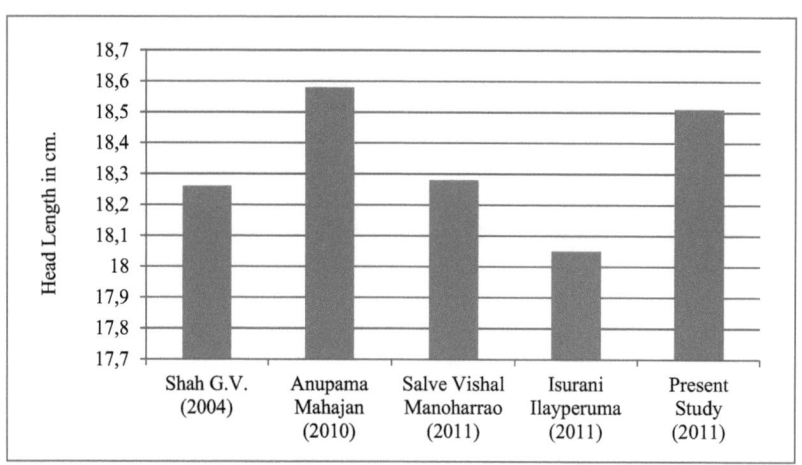

Table No. 9 - Comparison of present study with the other studies for head length of female students

Studies	Range	Mean
Shah G.V.	14.1 – 18.9	16.5
Anupama Mahajan	14.21 – 21.89	17.92
Salve Vishal Manohar	16.3 – 19.1	17.26
Isurani Ilayperuma	–	17.5
Present Study	14.40 – 19.50	17.53

Bar diagram showing comparison of present study with the other studies for head length of female students

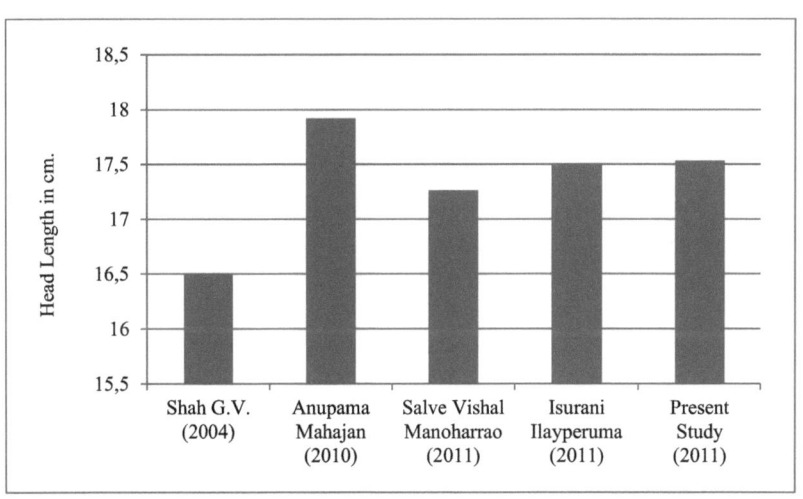

Table No. 10 - Comparison of present study with the other studies for head breadth of male students

Studies	Range	Mean
Shah G.V.	12.7 – 16.4	14.56
Anupama Mahajan	12.03 – 17.92	15.68
Salve Vishal Manohar	13.2 – 14.4	13.82
Isurani Ilayperuma	–	14.78
Present Study	13.0 – 16.40	14.63

Bar diagram showing comparison of present study with the other studies for head breadth of male students

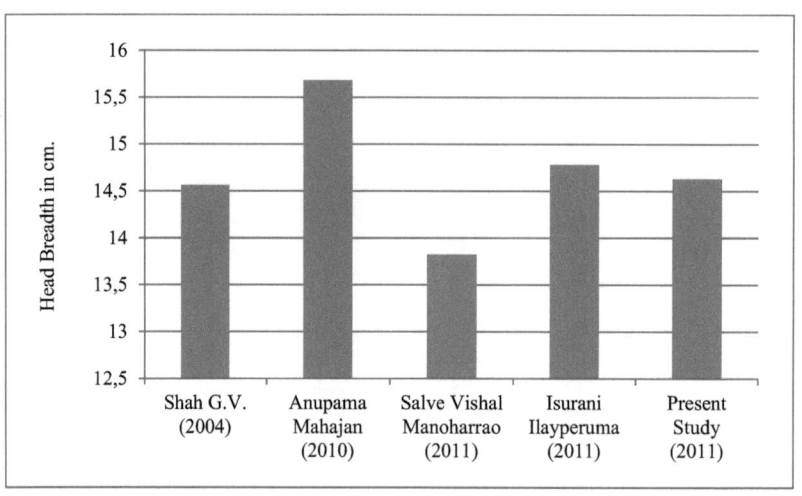

Table No. 11 - Comparison of present study with the other studies for head breadth of female students

Studies	Range	Mean
Shah G.V.	12.7 – 15.6	14.1
Anupama Mahajan	12.02 – 17.67	14.72
Salve Vishal Manohar	12.8 – 14.3	13.49
Isurani Ilayperuma	–	14.11
Present Study	13.10 – 16.50	14.32

Bar diagram showing comparison of present study with the other studies for head breadth of female students

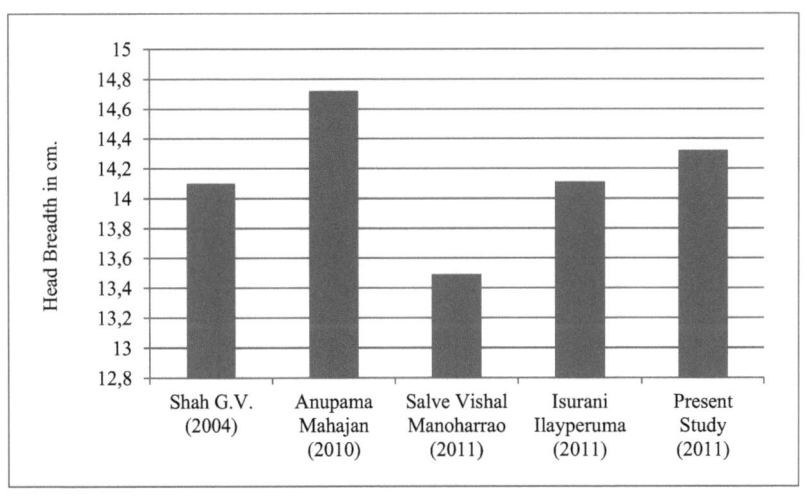

Table No. 12 - Comparison of present study with the other studies for cephalic index of male students

Studies	Range	Mean
Shah G.V.	71.01 – 90.0	80.42
Anupama Mahajan	71.01 – 92.0	81.34
Salve Vishal Manohar	69.11 – 79.33	75.68
Isurani Ilayperuma	–	78.04
Present Study	68.50 – 88.34	79.15

Bar diagram showing comparison of present study with the other studies for cephalic index of male students

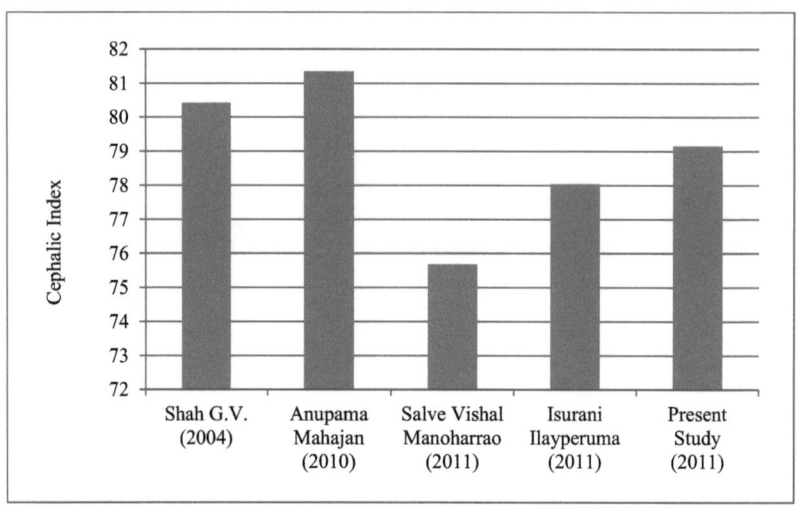

Table No. 13 - Comparison of present study with the other studies for cephalic index of female students

Studies	Range	Mean
Shah G.V.	72.01 – 89.0	81.20
Anupama Mahajan	71.01 – 92.0	85.75
Salve Vishal Manohar	71.67 – 84.52	78.20
Isurani Ilayperuma	–	79.32
Present Study	72.43 – 90.62	81.66

Bar diagram showing comparison of present study with the other studies for cephalic index of female students

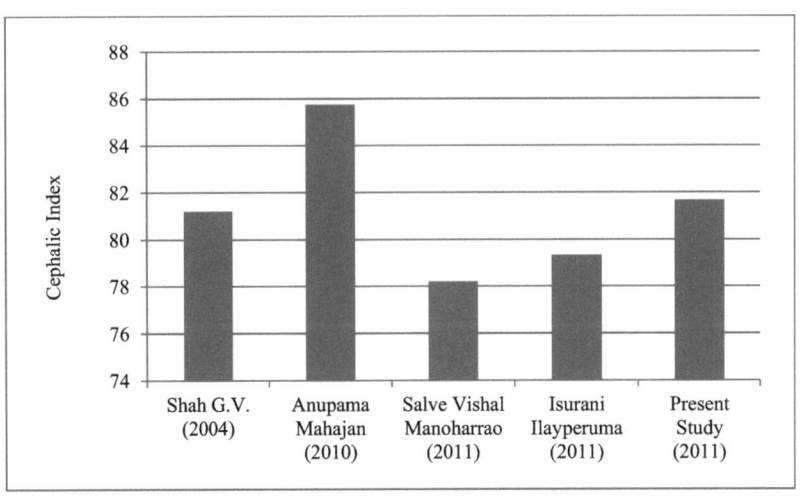

Table No. 14 - Comparison of present study with the other studies for cephalic index

Studies	Range	Mean
Shah G.V.	71.10 – 89.77	80.81
Anupama Mahajan	71.02 – 91.56	85.53
Salve Vishal Manohar	69.11 – 84.52	76.94
Isurani Ilayperuma	–	78.54
Present Study	68.50 – 90.62	80.41

Bar diagram showing comparison of present study with the other studies for cephalic index

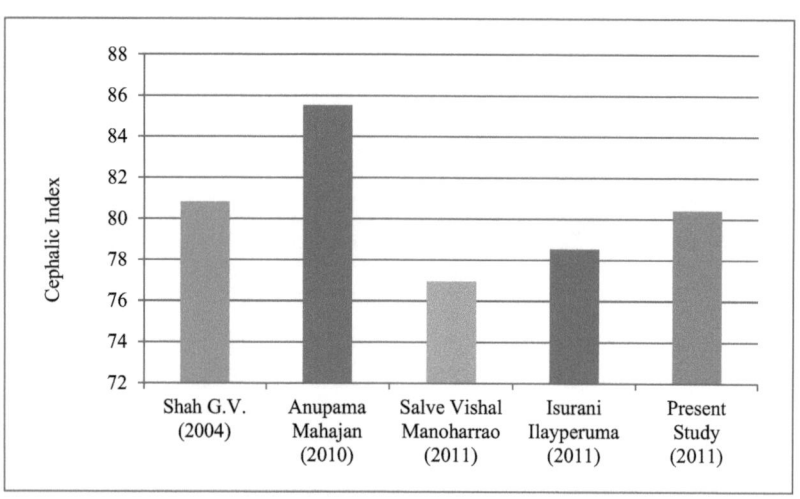

CONCLUSION

Racial variations in the cranium were recorded. Variations in cephalic indices between and within populations have been attributed to a complex interaction between genetic and environmental factors.[22]

The result of the present study shows that majority of male (191 out of 400) and female students (296 out of 400) are brachycephalic. The mean Cephalic index of both the sex (80.41) also shows the brachycephalisation of the population, which is also considered to be an important parameter for more towards civilization.

The current study and its statistical analysis conforms with the observation of previous workers and the range also falls within the normal mean parameters mentioned in the past.

Observing the tables and graphs it can be implied that the values of present study coincide with the values as observed in the previous studies.

The present study also get strengthened by previous work of G.V. shah in Gujarat, by Anupama Mahajan in Punjab and by Isurani Hayperuma in sri Lanka which shows brachycepalic dominancy in population in this region of southeast continent.

This data can be useful for forensic medicine experts, plastic surgeons, anatomist, anthropologist, oral surgeons and for clinical and research purposes.

The Important conclusions that can be drawn are as follows:

1. Cephalic index is an important parameter for deciding the race and sex of an individual whose identity is unknown.

2. A large body of evidence shows a clear racial variation in cephalic index. Therefore detailed knowledge of the population specific data on biometric features of the cranium is important.

3. The Index is important in comparison of the crania of populations from different racial backgrounds, assessing growth and development of an individual and in the diagnosis of any abnormalities of cranial size and shape.

4. Brachycephalisation is an evidence of continuous growth of brain more in the lateral direction.

BIBLIOGRAPHY

1. El-Feghi I, Sid-Ahmad MA & Ahmadi M. Automatic localization of craniofacial landmarks for assisted Cephalometry. *Pattern Recognition, 37*:609 - 21, 2004.

2. Grau V, Alcaniz M, Juan MC, Monserrat C & Knoll C. Automatic localization of Cephalometry landmarks. *J. of Biomedical Informatics, 34*:146 - 56, 2001.

3. Rao NG. Text Book of Forensic Medicine & Toxicology. 2nd edition.2010, Japee brothers Medical Publisher (P) Ltd.93-94.

4. Hrdlicka Ales, Anthropomery, published by - The Wistab Institute of Anatomy and Biology, Philadelphia. 1920, pp. : 7,14.

5. Shah GV, Jadhav HR. The study of cephalic index in students of Gujarat. Journal of Anatomical society of India 2004; 53(1):25-6.

6. Singh Vishram, Anatomy of head neck and brain, 2011, 1st Edn., Mosby,

Saunders, Churchill Livingstone, Butterworth Heinemann & Hanley & Belfus are the health science imprints of Elsevier; pp. : 25.

7. Williams, P.; Dyson, M.; Dussak, J. E.; Bannister, L. H.; Berry, M.M.; Collins, P. & Ferguson, M. W. J.. *Grays Anatomy*, 1995, 38th Ed., Elsevier Churchill Livingstone, London; P: 607 – 612.

8. Raveendranath V. & Manjunath K. Y.; An anthropometric study of correlation between cephalic index, cranial volume and cranial measurements in Indian cadavers; *Indian Science Abstracts*; Sep. 2010: vol. 15 (ii); pp. – 55-58.

9. Rajesh Bardale, Principles of Forensic Medicine and Toxicology, 1st ed. Jaypee Brothers Medical Publishers, 2011, pp. : 40 – 41.

10. Reddy Narayan K.S.; The Essentials of forensic medicine and toxicology; 19th ed. 2000; Jaypee Brothers; pp. – 92.

11. Vishal Manoharrao Salve, Naga Raghunandan Thota, Anupama Patibandla. The Study Of Cephalic Index Of Andhra Region (India), Asian Journal of Medical Sciences 2 (2011) 53-55.

12. Ilayperuma Isurani , Evaluation of Cephalic Indices: A Clue for Racial and Sex Diversity, Int. J. Morphol., 29(1):112-117, 2011.

13. Anitha. M.R, Vijayanath.V, Raju .G.M, Vijayamahantesh S.N., Cephalic Index of North Indian Population, Anatomica Karnataka, Vol-5, (1) Page 40-43 (2011).

14. Bharati, S., Som, S., Bharati, P. and Vasulu, T. (2001), Climate and head form in India. *American Journal of Human Biology*, 13: 626–634.

15. Shah GV, Jadhav HR. The study of cephalic index in students of Gujarat. Journal of Anatomical society of India 2004; 53(1):25-6.

16. **Hossain Golam M. D., Lestrel Pete E. and Ohtsuki Fumio;** Secular changes in head dimensions of japanese adult male students over eight decades. *Homo – journal of comparative human biology* volume 55, issue 3, pages 239-250.

17. Lobo SW, Chandrasekhar TS, Kumar S; Cephalic index of Gurung community of Nepal - an anthropometric study; *Kathmandu Univ. Med J (KUMJ)*. 2005 Jul-Sep; 3(3):263-5.

18. Golalipour, M. J. The effect of ethnic factor on cephalic index in 17-20 years old females of North of Iran. Int. J. Morphol.,*24(3)*:319-322, 2006.

19. Zahra Vojdani, Soghra Bahmanpour, Shahla Momeni, Atieh Vasaghi, Azadeh Yazdizadeh, Amirali Karamifar, Amirhosseine Najafifar, Shahram Setoodehmaram & Ali Mokhtar, Cephalometry in 14-18 Years Old Girls and Boys of Shiraz-Iran High School; *Int. J. Morphol.,* 27(1):101-104, 2009.

20. Oladipo G.S., Olotu J.E., Suleiman Y., Anthropometric Studies of Cephalic Indices of the Ogonis in Nigeria, Asian Journal of Medical Sciences 1(2): 15- 17, 2009.

21. Odokuma, E. I., Akpuaka, F. C.2, Igbigbi, P. S., Otuaga, P. O. and Ejebe, D., Patterns of cephalic indexes in three West African populations, African Journal of Biotechnology Vol. 9(11), pp. 1658-1662, 15 March, 2010.

22. Mahajan A, Khurana BS, Batra APS. The study of cephalic index in Punjab students. Journal of Punjab Academy of Forensic Medicine & Toxicology. 2009; 9(2): 15-17.

23. Oladipo G.S., Okoh P.D. and Isong E.E., An anthropometric Studies of Cephalic Length, Cephalic Breadth and Cephalic Indices of the Ibibios of Nigeria, Asian Journal of Medical Sciences 2(3): 104-106, 2010.

24. Raveendranath V. , Manjunath K. Y., An anthropometric study of correlation between cephalic index, cranial volume and cranial measurements in indian cadavers, Indian science abstracts, vol.15, No(II), Sep.- 2010, (55-8).

25. Adejuwon S.A., Salawu O.T., Eke C.C, Femi-Akinlosotu W. and Odaibo A.B.; A Craniometric Study of Adult Humans Skulls from Southwestern Nigeria, Asian Journal of Medical Sciences 3(1): 23-25, 2011.

26. Jadav H. R ., Kariya V.B. , Kodiyatar B. B. ,Pesi C.A, A Study to Correlate Cephalic Index Of Various Caste/Races Of Gujarat State, NJIRM 2011; Vol. 2(2).April-June.

27. M.B. Maina, O. Mahdi and G.D. Kalayi. Study of Vertical and Transverse Cephalic Indices in Three Ethnic Groups of North-eastern Nigerian Origin. *Trends in Applied Sciences Research*, 6: 1280-1286.

28. Anitha. M.R, Vijayanath.V, Raju .G.M, Vijayamahantesh S.N., Cephalic Index of North Indian Population, Anatomica Karnataka, Vol-5, (1) Page 40-43 (2011).

29. Salve Manoharrao Vishal , Thota Raghunandan Naga , Patibandla Anupama, The Study Of Cephalic Index Of Andhra Region (India), Asian Journal of Medical Sciences 2 (2011) 53-55.

30. Hrdlicka Ales, Anthropomery, published by - The Wistab Institute of Anatomy and Biology, Philadelphia. 1920, pp. : 55 - 57.

31. Hrdlicka Ales, Anthropomery, published by - The Wistab Institute of Anatomy and Biology, Philadelphia. 1920, pp. : 68 - 72.

32. Hrdlicka Ales, Anthropomery, published by - The Wistab Institute of Anatomy and Biology, Philadelphia. 1920, pp. : 151.